YOUR KNOWLEDGE HAS VALUE

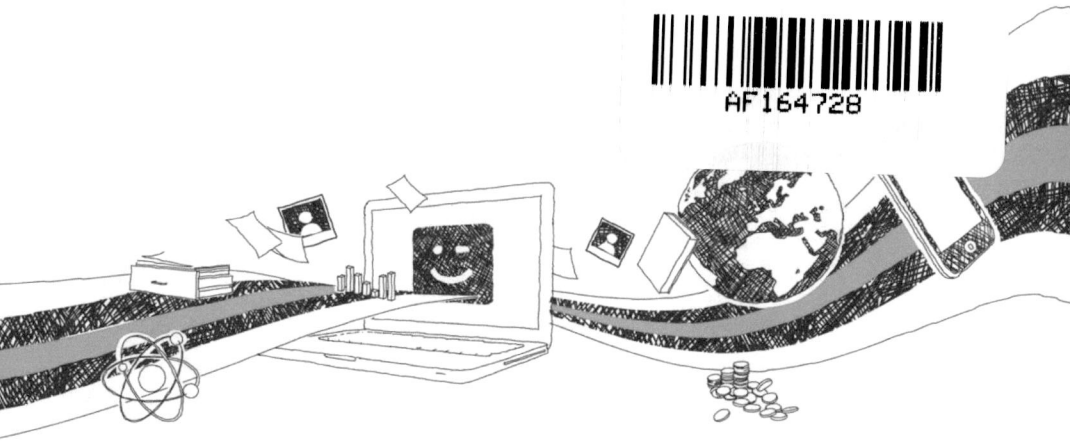

- We will publish your bachelor's and master's thesis, essays and papers

- Your own eBook and book - sold worldwide in all relevant shops

- Earn money with each sale

Upload your text at www.GRIN.com
and publish for free

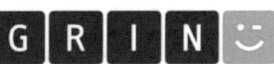

Bibliographic information published by the German National Library:

The German National Library lists this publication in the National Bibliography; detailed bibliographic data are available on the Internet at http://dnb.dnb.de .

This book is copyright material and must not be copied, reproduced, transferred, distributed, leased, licensed or publicly performed or used in any way except as specifically permitted in writing by the publishers, as allowed under the terms and conditions under which it was purchased or as strictly permitted by applicable copyright law. Any unauthorized distribution or use of this text may be a direct infringement of the author s and publisher s rights and those responsible may be liable in law accordingly.

Imprint:

Copyright © 2017 GRIN Verlag, Open Publishing GmbH
Print and binding: Books on Demand GmbH, Norderstedt Germany
ISBN: 9783668576650

This book at GRIN:

http://www.grin.com/en/e-book/381254/liver-congestion-causes-chronic-fatigue

Patrick Kimuyu

Liver Congestion Causes Chronic Fatigue

GRIN Publishing

GRIN - Your knowledge has value

Since its foundation in 1998, GRIN has specialized in publishing academic texts by students, college teachers and other academics as e-book and printed book. The website www.grin.com is an ideal platform for presenting term papers, final papers, scientific essays, dissertations and specialist books.

Visit us on the internet:

http://www.grin.com/

http://www.facebook.com/grincom

http://www.twitter.com/grin_com

Liver Congestion Causes Chronic Fatigue

Name: Patrick K. Kimuyu

Table of Content

Table of Content 2
Abstract 2
Introduction 4
Liver Congestion and Chronic Fatigue 5
Stress and Liver Congestion 9
Herbal Remedies 10
Consequences of Retoxification Reactions 11
Conclusion 12
References 14

Abstract

    Liver congestion is becoming an epidemic condition whose health consequences seem to be unbearable. Currently, humans are living in toxic environments, especially with regard to dietary sources, which are coupled with unhealthy lifestyle.

    Liver is involved in disease conditions to restore normal cellular activity. Therefore, any impairment of the liver functions leads to detrimental outcomes although direct symptoms are not manifested at the onset of the liver dysfunctions. This situation is worsened by the complexity of liver diagnosis. In most cases, liver problems are not easily detectable with routine diagnosis procedures.

There are several principal causes of liver congestion. First, liver congestion may be caused by toxins accumulation in the liver leading to overload which means that the liver is unable to clear toxins from the body. From a physiological perspective, excessive intake of noxious substances in the blood circulation causes physiological imbalances of various components including PH and nutrients availability for the cells.

In addition, diet causes liver toxicity when it contains numerous food additives and dietary toxins, primarily iron, which is contained in most processed foods such as white bread. These additives facilitate crystallization in the liver cells which, in turn leads to formation of salt deposits in the bile stream.

Chronic fatigue syndrome is worsened by liver congestion because hormonal imbalances serve as some of the most principal contributors to the occurrence of CFS. Therefore, one of the most reliable approaches of managing CFS is through the enhancement of the liver function.

On the other hand, stress serves as a trigger and an ongoing feeder of physiological imbalances; thus, it contributes to liver congestion and chronic fatigue.

There are several approaches of addressing liver congestion including liver flushes and cleanses, but herbal remedies such as vegetable juicing and milk thistle are the most reliable alternatives because they are not associated with retoxification reactions.

Introduction

Liver congestion is becoming an epidemic condition whose health consequences seem to be unbearable. Currently, humans are living in toxic environments, especially with regard to dietary sources, which are coupled with unhealthy lifestyle. As a result, some body organs and tissues are experiencing immense challenging in maintaining the body's normal physiology through homeostatic regulation of various fluids and solutes. In theory, the functioning of all body organs depends on the physiological conditions in the body. At some point, their functions are diminished whereas favorable or rather normal physiological conditions enhance normal functioning. Ideally, an individual's body is said to be normal and healthy when all biological processes and organs are functioning normally under optimal physiological conditions. Therefore, any deviation from normal conditions is usually accompanied with a characteristic biological abnormality. In most cases, diseases are caused by microorganisms such as bacteria, viruses and fungus. However, it is worth noting that, not all microorganisms cause diseases. Indeed, some microorganisms are quite useful for the normal biological functions of the human body. For instance, the so-called normal micro flora contribute to an individual's health in one way or the other, especially in maintaining microbial balance in the digestive and reproductive systems. On the other hand, deviation from the normal state may be caused by physiological imbalances or deficiencies of essential body requirements, and this is the phenomenon associated with liver congestion. Therefore, this paper will provide a comprehensive review of liver congestion and its relation to chronic fatigue. In addition, it will discuss the role of stress in liver congestion as one of the most principal causes. Moreover, it will provide an overview on the liver congestion remedies and the consequences of liver flushes or cleanses and acupuncture.

Liver Congestion and Chronic Fatigue

It is believed that, liver congestion has a close link to virtually all recurrent illnesses because the liver plays a very pivotal role in functioning and growth of all cells in the body. It is also involved in disease conditions to restore normal cellular activity. Therefore, any impairment of the liver functions leads to detrimental outcomes although direct symptoms are not manifested at the onset of the liver dysfunctions. This situation is worsened by the complexity of liver diagnosis. In most cases, liver problems are not easily detectable with routine diagnosis procedures. For instance, liver stones, which are the principal causes of liver congestion, are difficult to detect using X-rays and ultrasound technologies (Scott, 2013). As a result, most people live with liver congestion for quite a long time before it is detected; only when devastating damage of the organ has already occurred; thus conventional medicine does not help in managing the condition.

From a biological perspective, the liver is one of the most vital organs in the body without which physiological processes such as chemical balances cannot occur when its functions are impaired. In reality, the human liver is believed to be involved in more than 500 body functions. Some of its functions include biosynthesis of some macromolecules such as cholesterol which is used by the body in forming cellular membranes, hormones and bile (Wilson, 2013). It is also responsible for the manufacture of non-essential amino acids which serve as building blocks for the synthesis of proteins. In addition, it is involved in storage of vitamins and some mineral elements in the body. Moreover, it helps in recycling of iron by breaking down hemoglobin in old red blood cells and converts polyporpyrin components of hemoglobin into bile salts, which aid the digestion of lipids.

On the other hand, liver plays a pivotal biological role in the elimination of toxic substances from the body by converting them into water soluble byproducts for excretion. As such, it plays a detoxification role in the body in which poisons and wastes are converted into non-toxic compounds for transportation to excretion systems such as the kidneys and sweat glands. In theory, it filters blood of noxious substances such as pesticides, fertilizers and other chemicals which are acquired from the environment through diet in which the detoxified substances are conveyed to the excretory systems through the bile stream (Scott, 2013). In case, the bile stream is blocked as a result of the formation of liver stones, most physiological functions of the liver are interrupted leading to a disease condition which is manifested as tiredness. In most cases, liver overload with toxins causes liver congestion in which its detoxification capabilities diminish. It is also worth noting that unfiltered blood is thick compared to filtered blood, which is produced by a healthy liver. As a result, congested liver is characterized by impaired blood flow in the bile stream even when liver stones are not present (Chang, 2012). This causes abnormal functioning of the body, primarily due to the lack of liver hormones and proteins which controls the way the body grow, function and heal. Ideally, this is how the liver affects the health of cells leading to chronic illnesses owing to liver congestion and chronic fatigue syndrome is one of unhealthy conditions.

Ordinarily, there are several principal causes of liver congestion. First, liver congestion may be caused by toxins accumulation in the liver leading to overload which means that the liver is unable to clear toxins from the body. From a physiological perspective, excessive intake of noxious substances in the blood circulation causes physiological imbalances of various components including PH and nutrients availability for the cells (Pitts, 2013). Therefore, physiological imbalances, primarily in regard to PH facilitate crystallization of different chemical compounds in the liver leading to deposition of salts in the bile stream. This deposition of crystallized salts is what causes the hardening and blockage of bile ducts; a characteristic condition referred to as gall stones, which are responsible for liver congestion. In addition, failure of the liver to filter wastes and toxic substances from the blood for elimination leads to excessive accumulation of toxins in the body which cause physiological imbalances and cellular toxicity.

On the other hand, dietary regime and lifestyle changes form the second cause of liver congestion. Liver is involved in the processing of some dietary components, primarily carbohydrates. It has been found that liver regulates blood glucose through two main biological processes, namely; gluconeogenesis and glycolysis. It is believed that, excessive intake of carbohydrates causes changes in blood PH leading to reduced activity of liver cells. This causes an increase of blood glucose beyond the normal range and interferes with the normal liver functioning leading to the hindrance of all other biological processes in the liver (Pitts, 2013). Therefore, irregular blood glucose levels causes liver congestion, which is manifested through feeling of the general body weakness or jaundice, especially when bile ducts are blocked by gallstones.

Diet may also cause liver toxicity when it contains numerous food additives and dietary toxins, primarily iron, which is contained in most processed foods such as white bread (Wilson, 2013). These additives facilitate crystallization in the liver cells which, in turn leads to the formation of salt deposits in the bile stream. In addition, excessive alcohol intake causes liver toxicity because it is involved in alcohol breakdown into its byproducts. In some cases, alcohol increase in alcohol levels in the blood is caused by the fermentation of dietary components in the gastrointestinal tract in which acetaldehyde and other toxins are formed. Therefore, high levels of acetaldehyde cause liver toxicity because they lower blood PH leading to a significant decrease in liver functioning. However, it is worth noting that formation of toxins in the body may be caused by indigestion problems such as constipation in which microbial activities produce toxins after prolonged retention of food components in the bowel (Wilson, 2013).

Other causes of liver toxicity include overuse of drugs and nutrient deficiencies. Ideally, conventional medicine involves the use of drugs for treatment of diseases, ranging from infectious to non-communicable diseases. All drugs are toxic; thus, detoxification in the liver prevents the accumulation of toxic byproducts of over-the-counter or medical drugs. In chronic illnesses, these drugs are consumed for a long period leading to gradual accumulation toxic compounds in the body which cause liver congestion. This is the reason as to why alternative medicine serves as a reliable remedy for most illnesses, which require prolonged long term administration of conventional drugs to reduce liver toxicity. In regard to nutrient deficiencies, liver requires several dietary components such as zinc, chromium, vitamin C and selenium for detoxification processes (Wilson, 2013). Therefore, inadequate supply of these nutrients from the diet leads to abnormalities in liver functioning, which are attributable to liver congestion.

It is believed liver congestion causes devastating consequences on patients suffering from Chronic Fatigue Syndrome (CFS). Despite the controversy surrounding the possible causes of CFS, research reveals that this condition which is characterized with insomnia and general discomfort even after sleep or rest, is caused by hormonal imbalance, impaired immune system, trauma and psychiatric problems such as depression, stress and mental exhaustion. Genetic factors have also been found to play a significant role in the occurrence of CFS because it appears to run along family lines (NHS, 2013). In theory, glandular fever is believed to trigger CFS.

Chronic fatigue syndrome is worsened by liver congestion because hormonal imbalances serve as some of the most principal contributors to the occurrence of CFS. On the other hand, liver congestion causes impairment of carbohydrate metabolism leading to energy shortages in the cells. For instance, decrease in blood glucose level cannot be restored through glucose release from the liver cells because they are poisoned with wastes and toxins. As a result, lack of adequate energy supply in the body causes weakness of the body. In some cases, CFS patients are unable to engage in physical activity because energy reserves in their active muscles are depleted.

Therefore, one of the most reliable approaches of managing CFS is through the enhancement of the liver function. This ensures the maintenance of normal blood glucose levels. From a physiological perspective, proper functioning of the liver facilitates the conversion of glucose for storage whenever its levels are elevated to prevent a phenomenon referred to as Specific Dynamic Action (SDA) or heat increment which is experienced after a heavy carbohydrate meal. The fact that surges in temperature causes severity of CFS implies that uncontrolled glucose flow in the circulation, owing to the inability of the liver to lower glucose concentration in blood after meals worsens the condition.

Stress and Liver Congestion

On the other, stress triggers physiological imbalances, which are witnessed in liver congestion and chronic fatigue. Research studies indicate that stress causes low-grade fever n CFS patients. Ordinarily, stress activates the sympathetic nervous system which influences temperature regulation in the body through thermogenesis (Oka et al, 2013). In most cases, stress increases body temperature by decreasing catecholamine levels in the blood circulation while increasing the concentration of stress hormones such as cortisol. It has been found out that excessive stimulation of the adrenal glands to produce cortisol under continual stress episodes leads to an increase of cortisol beyond healthy levels, and this is believed to be responsible for the onset of metabolic syndrome. In metabolic syndrome, the liver is over stimulated to produce excessive levels of cholesterol which may cause heart problems (Livlong, 2013). It is also believed that stress enhances physiological imbalances by impairing with proper liver functioning. This occurs when excess cholesterol decreases blood flow in bile stream. As a result, blood does not leave the liver efficiently for cleansing of toxins, and wastes and this is also another cause of liver congestion.

Herbal Remedies

Liver congestion can be addressed with herbal remedies, rather than conventional medical approaches. Currently, there are several herbal remedies for liver congestion. For instance, vegetable juicing has proven to be helpful in enhancing liver functioning. Ordinarily, vegetables contain phytochemicals which act as antioxidants. Therefore, frequent intake of vegetable juices ensures adequate supply of antioxidants which aid in removing toxins from the body.

On the other hand, herbs such as milk thistle, turmeric, dandelion and globe artichoke play pivotal roles in enhancing the activity of liver cells. Milk thistle contains silymarin which acts a potent liver-protective agent. It boosts liver functioning in two principal ways. First, it facilitates rejuvenation of liver cells through stimulating protein synthesis which increases the production of new liver cells (Moritz, 2007). Therefore, damaged liver cells are frequently replaced with new ones; thus, maintaining normal liver functioning which relieves symptoms of liver congestion. Secondly, milk thistle produces phytochemicals which inhibit free radicals from damaging liver cells (Jensen, 2000).

Dandelion root facilitates the cleansing activity of the liver by promoting kidney functioning. It also restores liver functioning because it is non-toxic that is the reason why it has always been used as a reliable remedy for liver congestion (Jensen, 2000).

On the other hand, cynarin and curcumin which are produced by globe artichoke and turmeric, respectively, have antioxidant activity; thus, liver-protective. They also promote lipid metabolism and lower blood cholesterol which interferes with blood flow in the bile stream during detoxifying processes in the liver (Jensen, 2000).

Consequences of Retoxification Reactions

Liver congestion is addressed through liver flushes and cleanses to remove toxins from the blood. In practice, cleansing of blood improves the functioning of body cells owing to the improved supply of nutrients and clearance of wastes. Cleansing ensures efficient flow of blood in the bile stream and facilitates digestion through removing gallstones, which block the flow of bile fluid into the gut for lipid digestion (Richards, 2013).

On the other hand, acupuncture helps in addressing numerous physiological imbalances associated with liver congestion. For instance, medicinal herbs combined with acupuncture aid in discharging gallstones into the intestines for elimination from the body. It also prevents chronic fatigue through enhancing the functions of immune, digestive, circulatory and nervous systems. As such, it eliminates some adverse conditions involved in liver congestion (San Francisco Clinic, 2011).

However, it is worth noting that acupuncture, liver flushes and cleanses may have devastating consequences in individuals whose bodies are weak owing to retoxification reactions. Ordinarily, liver flushes and cleanses removes toxins and wastes from the body, but they do not establish efficient immune system activity. In addition, some of these approaches do not restore normal liver functioning through the replacement of damaged cells or introducing liver-protective mechanisms. Therefore, retoxification occurs shortly after liver flushes and cleanses, especially in weak individuals. This is the reason as to why alternative treatment remedies such as the use of herbs serves as the most reliable treatment option for liver congestion. Herbal remedies restores normal liver functioning and removes wastes and toxins from the body altogether. They also offer liver-protective mechanisms because most phyto-nutrients protect liver cells from being damaged by active radicals (Jensen, 2000).

Conclusion

Conclusively, liver congestion is linked to most chronic illnesses because the liver influences the function of all body cells. For instance, it promotes the production of amino acids which are used in the production of cellular proteins and hormones. Therefore, impairment of liver functioning causes physiological imbalances in the body leading the feeling of tiredness which is also a principal characteristic of chronic fatigue syndrome. It is believed that liver congestion causes severity of chronic fatigue syndrome because it lowers hormonal balance and lipid metabolism in the body. Stress is also believed to be a trigger of chronic fatigue because it stimulates excessive production of cortisol which, in turn increases cholesterol production. High levels of cholesterol impair blood flow in bile stream leading to slow cleansing of blood in the liver.

However, liver congestion and chronic fatigue can be addressed using alternative medicine. Some of the most reliable herbs include dandelion, turmeric, globe artichoke and vegetable juicing. Liver flushes and cleansing can also relieve liver congestion although retoxification reactions may cause devastating consequences.

References

Chang, J. (2012). *Liver Functions, Liver Disease, and Liver Cleanse.* Retrieved from http://www.sensiblehealth.com/Journey-01.xhtml

Jensen, K. (2000). *A Little Help for the Liver.* Retrieved from http://www.alive.com/articles/view/16547/a_little_help_for_the_liver

Livlong (2013). *The Liver's Crucial Role in Weight Loss.* Retrieved from http://livlong.ca/374/the-livers-crucial-role-in-weight-loss

Moritz, A. (2007). *Timeless Secrets of Health and Rejuvenation.* Minneapolis, MN: Ener-Chi Wellness Center.

NHS (2013). *Causes of Chronic Fatigue Syndrome.* Retrieved from http://www.nhs.uk/Conditions/Chronic-fatigue-syndrome/Pages/Causes.aspx

Oka, T. et al. (2013). *Psychological Stress Contributed to The Development of Low-Grade Fever in a Patient With Chronic Fatigue Syndrome: A Case Report.* Retrieved from http://www.bpsmedicine.com/content/7/1/7

Pitts, J. (2013). *What Causes a Congested Liver?* Retrieved from http://www.healthguidance.org/entry/11466/1/What-Causes-a-Congested-Liver.html

Richards, M. V. (2013). *Have You Had a Coffee Break Today? (But Not the Way You Think!).* eBookIt.com.

San Francisco Clinic (2011). *Acupuncture and Chinese Medicine.* Retrieved from http://www.chinese-medicine-works.com/san-francisco-acupuncture/conditions.html

Scott, T. (2013).*Liver Congestion, a Growing Epidemic.* Retrieved from http://www.thespiritualcatalyst.com/articles/liver-congestion-a-growing-epidemic

Wilson, L. (2013). *Liver Dysfunctions*. Retrieved from http://drlwilson.com/Articles/LIVER.HTM

YOUR KNOWLEDGE HAS VALUE

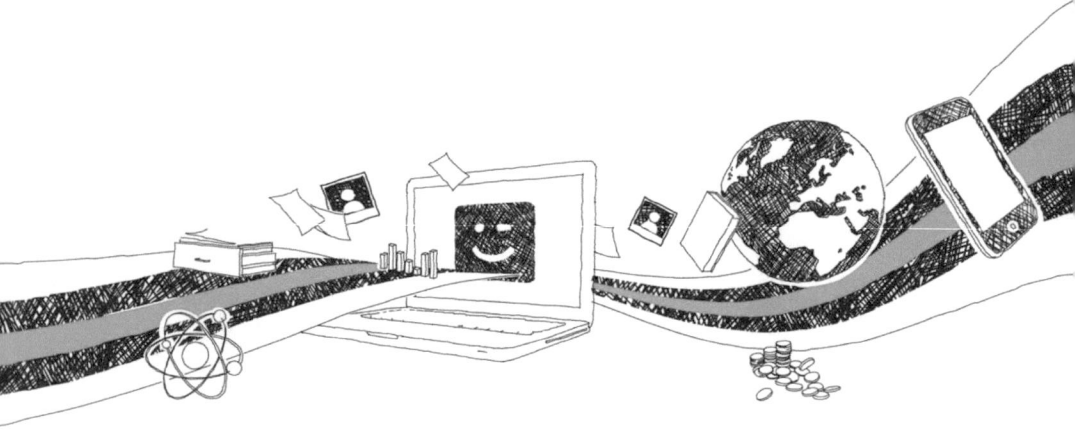

- We will publish your bachelor's and master's thesis, essays and papers

- Your own eBook and book - sold worldwide in all relevant shops

- Earn money with each sale

Upload your text at www.GRIN.com and publish for free

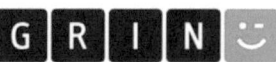